I0411343

Wheat Free Diet Benefits

By

Sherri Neal

ISBN-13: 978-1490590561

Table of Contents

Wheat Free Diet Benefits

By Sherri Neal

© Copyright 2013 Sherri Neal

First Published, 2013

Printed in the United States of America

Introduction

A wheat free diet is defined simply as a diet free from wheat or products made of wheat. This diet is based principally on the fact that wheat is a primary allergen and that it can cause allergies like celiac disease which is why the most basic principle of this diet is the avoidance of wheat in the diet or any products that contain wheat such as cakes, bread, etc. The wheat free diet is mostly applied by those who are on a gluten-free diet because wheat is known as food that contains gluten. Gluten is a component found in wheat and other grains that is known to cause many disorders including the celiac disease. This is why all who are on a gluten-free diet are most likely on a wheat-free diet as well.

But it is not only those who are on a gluten-free diet who applies the wheat free diet nowadays but also those who want to be healthy all over. Even if wheat has its own share of benefits especially to the health, your health can also benefit if you go on a wheat free diet. The question is, why? What are the benefits of a wheat free diet and why is this so popular? What can people, most especially dieters, get with the wheat free diet?

Wheat Free Diet Benefits

<u>Weight Loss</u>. Most people who want to lose weight because they are suffering from overweight or obesity can also benefit from wheat free diet as this diet is known to promote or contribute to weight loss. Wheat is a food product known to have high GI or glycaemic index which refers to how fast blood sugar levels rise. In other words, wheat contributes to making blood sugar levels raise fast and this can be a contributor to obesity. Wheat is also a product known to be a very potent appetite stimulant which can also contribute to overeating and gaining weight fast. But weight loss can be achieved through a wheat free diet since your GI won't be as high and your appetite will no longer be as high and as strong as before.

<u>Controlled and prevented diabetes</u>. Many diabetic patients and those who want to steer clear of diabetes also go on a wheat free diet because this type of diet is also known to be very effective in preventing and controlling diabetes. Diabetes is a disease known to be caused by high blood sugar levels and because wheat contains amylopectin A, a starch known to be converted easily to sugar in the blood,

it is also known to be a very potent cause of diabetes. And as mentioned, wheat has high GI which is also a contributor to making blood sugar levels raise fast, thereby contributing to the onset or worsening of diabetes. But you can prevent or control diabetes through a wheat free diet because you would be free from the amylopectin A and high GI and so, your blood sugar levels won't quickly rise.

Recovery from celiac disease. Celiac disease is a disease that is also known as an allergic reaction that triggers digestive problems like stomach ache, diarrhea, etc. Most people who are suffering from celiac disease are also applying the wheat free diet in their lives because this type of diet is also known to help a person recover from this disease. Why? Celiac disease is a disease that's mostly triggered by gluten which is why this is also often called a gluten allergy. Gluten can be found in wheat and so, wheat is known to be one of the major trigger factors of celiac disease along with other gluten-rich foods. Now, going on wheat free diet can help a person recover from celiac disease since they will no longer be consuming wheat and other foods made of wheat that contains gluten. In other words, your gluten allergy will no longer be triggered, making you recover from that disease successfully.

Treatment of digestive problems like ulcerative colitis, etc. It is not only celiac disease that's known to cause digestive problems but also ulcerative colitis. This disease is commonly known as a colon disease due to inflammation. Wheat has WGA lectin, a kind of protein that can cause inflammation in the stomach and intestines and can really cause ulcerative colitis as well as even trigger other digestive problems like diarrhea, constipation, etc. Those who are experiencing this disease and those who want to prevent this disease go on a wheat free diet. BY banning wheat from their diet, they are freeing themselves from this lectin that can cause gut inflammation and prevent ulcerative colitis and other digestive diseases. Through wheat free diet, you can benefit a lot of from a healthy digestive system from the stomach down to the intestines.

Blood Cholesterol improvement as well as prevention and recovery from heart diseases. Those who are suffering heart diseases due to high blood cholesterol levels also apply the wheat free diet in their lives. As mentioned, wheat is a food product that contains the starch called amylopectin A as well as wheat is also known to contain lectin WGA that may cause gut inflammation or leaky gut. Having high blood sugar levels can cause diabetes which can in turn, cause heart diseases due to high cholesterol levels as well and leaky gut us not only a disease that means inflamed gut but also a disease that may lead to heart disease. But when you go on a wheat free diet, you can be free from all the components found in wheat that are known to trigger high blood sugar and cholesterol levels that may contribute to heart disease.

Reduced risk of anemia and blood diseases. People suffering from anemia and other blood disease are also most likely to benefit from the wheat free diet. Wheat does not only contain components that increase the risk of diabetes, heart diseases, digestive problems, etc. but it is also a food product known to contain phytate. Phytate is a substance that can hamper the easy absorption of essential minerals like iron, zinc, etc. Now, iron is popularly known as a blood vitamin or in other words, it makes your blood healthy. When these minerals are absorbed well by the body, this results to prevention or treatment of anemia and other blood related diseases. But since wheat contains phytate, consumption of this food may hamper iron absorption and this may lead to anemia and other diseases. Through the wheat free diet, you will no longer consume wheat that has phytate which means that iron absorption can be performed by the body successfully already.

Foods to Avoid During Wheat Free Diet

When going on a wheat free diet, it is important to know some of the foods to avoid while on the diet. These are the foods that should never be consumed as they contain wheat or ingredients that come from wheat.

PASTRIES. These are the most common foods to avoid because they are mostly the foods that are breaded using wheat flour. This group of foods includes pies, cakes, doughnuts, pizzas, etc. Wheat is mostly the reason why diabetics are advised not to consume too much of these products aside from the fact that these pastries are mostly sweetened.

PROCESSED FOODS. Processed foods also contain flour that mostly comes from wheat. These types of foods include meatballs, luncheon meat, hotdogs, sausages, etc. This is because they are not purely meat but they contain flour as well.

PASTA AND NOODLES. This refers to pastas made of flour that contain wheat like chow mien, gnocchi, lo mein, macaroni, spaghetti, and a lot more. They are mostly commercially made pastas wherein wheat is their main ingredient. Any food or meal that contains these pastas and noodles should not be included during the wheat free diet.

BREADED FOODS. While on the wheat free diet, you can consume meat, poultry and other protein foods and vegetables as you like as long as they are not prepared with breading. In other words, breaded pork, breaded chicken, breaded fish and seafood like tempura, etc. should be avoided. Even if they are healthy foods, if they are prepared with wheat products, they should be avoided as much as possible.

SAUCES AND GRAVIES. Sauces and gravies may make any dish interesting and tasty but they should be avoided as well during the wheat free diet. This is because they most likely contain wheat from flours used to thicken the sauce. These causes and gravies include tomato sauce and any thickened sauce. While you are not advised to avoid sauce altogether, it just depends on whether the sauce you prepare is thickened or not.

All in all, you are to avoid foods containing wheat product as ingredients such as hydrolyzed vegetable protein, gelatinized starch, modified food starch and a lot more.

Best Foods to Include in Your Wheat Free Diet

If there are foods to avoid during the wheat free diet, there are also foods best included in your wheat free diet. These are the foods that contain no wheat and can help you achieve the benefits that a wheat free diet can offer.

FRUITS AND VEGETABLES. These are very good food items to include in your wheat free diet as they contain no wheat provided they are not prepared with breading and flour. While on the wheat free diet, you can include fruits and vegetables such as apples, squash, spinach, citrus fruits, asparagus, broccoli, berries, etc.

DAIRY. You can also consume dairy products during the wheat free diet provided they are gluten-free (if your purpose is to apply a gluten-free diet) such as milk, cottage cheese and sour cream or any dairy product provided they are not mixed with wheat products.

MEAT AND POULTRY. Eggs, beef, pork, chicken, fish, shrimp, etc. can also be included in your wheat free diet provided they are not prepared with the use of four and breading as well as they are not cooked in thickened sauce.

CANNED GOODS. You can also consume canned gods even if you are on a wheat free diet because there are processed and canned goods that contain no wheat such as tuna, canned beans, etc.

GRAINS AND PASTAS. Grains and pastas are not altogether banned as long as you are careful what to choose and include in your diet. You can incorporate rice, buckwheat, legumes, soy, and other types of grains. You can even include rye and other grains since they are not wheat as long as you are not on a gluten-free diet.

FLOURS. Being on a wheat free diet does not mean you can avoid the use of flour altogether. It just depends on what kind of flour you choose. While wheat flour is banned, you can incorporate almond flour, cassava flour, rice flour, etc. in your diet.

Wheat Free Diet Meal Plan

Knowing the foods to avoid as well as the foods to include in your wheat free diet makes it easy to whip up your very own wheat free diet meal plan. It is important to have wheat free diet meal plan as it is like preparing what you can have for breakfast, lunch, snack and dinner daily. When you have a meal plan, you can simply refer to this plan every time you shop and every time you prepare something for your every day meals. Preparing your every own wheat free diet meal plan is not that difficult as this diet is not too restrictive compared to other types of diet. The diet mainly bashes wheat and not other food items you love. With this, here is an example of a good wheat free diet meal plan that you can follow:

Breakfast

SET 1:

1 pc. Hard-boiled egg

1 serving of rice porridge

1 glass of milk

1 banana

SET 2:

1 fried egg

1 cup of rice/1 bowl of porridge

1 glass of milk

1 apple

SET 3:

1 bowl of Chex cereal

1 glass of milk

1 banana

SET 4:

Bacon and eggs

Bread made of rice flour

A glass of milk

1 serving of wheat free yogurt

SET 5:

1 toast (bread made of other types of flour other than

wheat flour)

2 slices of cottage cheese

1 glass of orange juice

1 apple

Lunch

SET 1:

1 cup of rice

1 pc of steak

1 cup of asparagus

1 glass of orange juice

1 cup of berries

SET 2:

1 cup of brown rice

1 pc of salmon

1 cup of spinach

A glass of water

1 orange

SET 3:

1 sandwich (consisting of bread made of rice flour, tuna, tomatoes, greens, cottage cheese)

1 glass of lemon juice

1 banana

SET 4:

1 Chicken sandwich (rice flour bread, chicken, tomatoes, lettuce, onions,)
1 glass of iced tea
1 orange

SET 5:

1 cup of rice
1 lobster
1 cup of lettuce
1 glass of water
1 slice of pineapple

Snacks

SET 1:

1 cup of almond nuts

1 glass of milk

SET 2:

1 cup of dried fruit

I glass of water

SET 3:

1 serving of fruits salad

I glass of orange juice

SET 4:

1 bowl of popcorn

1 glass of lemon juice

SET 5:

1 serving of fruit yogurt (no additives)

A glass of water

SET 6:

1 toast made of bread baked with other flours

1 slice of cottage cheese

1 glass of fruit juice

SET 7:

1 slice of wheat free cassava cake

1 glass of milk or tea

Dinner

SET 1:

1 cup of mashed potatoes

1 pc of steamed salmon

1 cup of steamed vegetables

1 glass of water

1 pc of orange

SET 2:

1 serving of sweet potatoes

1 serving of ground turkey

1 serving of roasted vegetables

1 glass of orange juice

1 cup of fruit mix

SET 3:

1 cup of brown rice

Stir fried vegetables

1 cup of sautéed shrimp

1 glass of lemon iced tea

1 pc of banana

SET 4:

1 cup of brown rice

1 pc of steamed chicken

1 cup of broccoli

1 glass of water

1 apple

It is up to you to follow this wheat free diet meal plan or you create your own meal plan.

How to Start Reaping The Wheat Free Diet Benefits

<u>Get in touch with your wheat free diet purpose</u>. If you want to start reaping the wheat free diet benefits, first, you must know what your purpose for dieting is. You will not reach your goal if you have no idea why you are dieting wheat free.

If you are dieting for weight loss, consider other food items that should be avoided aside from the wheat free food items.

If you are wheat free dieting for recovery from celiac disease, you should also start being watchful of gluten in your diet.

If you know what your purpose is, you will know how to further improve your diet plan so that it would benefit your wheat free diet purpose.

<u>Get to know more about the basic principles of the wheat free diet</u>. Research and study more to get to know more

about the wheat free diet. It's not enough to go on a wheat free diet just because it is not too restrictive.

In your research, read reviews about this type of diet to know more about it especially if the reviews and testimonials are from readers who have applied this diet already. There are lots of resources where you can gather wheat free diet information.

You can also ask experts or professional help if you want to get more accurate information.

Bear in mind the foods to avoid and foods to include. Before you start reaping the benefits, it is a must to bear in mind the foods that you need to avoid and the foods best for the wheat free diet. You will never reap the benefits of a wheat free diet if you fail in avoiding the banned foods.

First, make a list of the foods you need to avoid whether it is a shopping list or just a note. Make sure that it goes along well with your dieting purpose.

Second, gather wheat free diet recipes or recipes that only include the foods best for wheat free diet.

This step will help you fill your shopping cart and your fridge with the right food items only.

Create a wheat free diet meal plan. Before you start the wheat free diet, create your wheat free diet meal plan first. This will save you time thinking of what sort of meal you are going to prepare every day. It is up to you to follow other wheat free diet meal plans or create your own as long as you abide by the right food items to include and to avoid.

Set your goal. This is the duration by which you are going to be on a wheat free diet. How many weeks do you want to have your wheat free diet? Mark it on your calendar. This step is only for those who are trying to lose weight. The wheat free diet may be advised for long term only for those people who are really allergic to wheat.

Wheat Free Diet Cons and Side Effects

If there are wheat free diet benefits, there are also some wheat free diet cons and side effects that you must be aware of. Knowing these side effects and cons can help you avoid them and make sure that despite their existence, you are still reaping the benefits of a wheat free diet.

Low energy. This is one of the most common side effects of a wheat free diet. Wheat free dieters experience this because a wheat free diet deprives nutrients and minerals that wheat can offer such as carbohydrates and energy. You may experience weakness and lack of vigor. Wheat is a good source of energy and if this is not incorporated in the diet, expect to have low energy during your diet days.

Folic Acid Deficiency. The wheat free diet may not be advisable for pregnant women who are in dire need of folic acid. Folic acid is very essential as this prevents birth defects as it contributes to the healthy development of the baby. Wheat and wheat products are known to be rich sources of folic acid and so without the consumption of wheat, the wheat freed diet can be dangerous for pregnant women.

Extreme weight loss. The wheat free diet is a very effective weight loss diet; however, it could lead to extreme weight loss if you don't mind the calories you take in. Without wheat and wheat products in the diet, you will experience low caloric intake and this can result to weight loss. Even if this is what your primary purpose is, since too much weight loss can have ill effects to your health, the wheat free diet may be harmful for your health as well.

The wheat free diet may have its share of cons and side effects but these side effects and cons are only minor cons and effects. In other words, these can be avoided. You can reap the wheat freed diet benefits without having to go through or experience the cons and side effects. You only need to abide by some very helpful tips to help you control the side effects of the wheat free diet.

Helpful Tips to Achieve the Wheat Free Diet Benefits

<u>Do not ignore the labels</u>. If you are going to buy or shop for food items while on a wheat free diet, make sure you always check the labels so that you can always ensure that what you are eating is wheat free. You must be aware of the various ingredients that the food items should contain before you buy them. Get to know the ingredients that contain wheat and always check the labels to ensure that these wheat ingredients are not contained in that product before you buy it. By not ignoring the labels, you can always ensure that you are buying the right wheat free food items during your wheat free diet.

<u>Increase your carbohydrate intake from other carb sources</u>. Since carbohydrates is an essential nutrient that can help your body get the energy it needs every day, you need to ensure that you are getting the normal amount of carbohydrates daily. Since the wheat free diet can deprive you of this, you need to increase your intake of other food sources that are rich in carbohydrates aside from wheat. This is so that you can still be energized even if you are on

a wheat free diet. Some food items that are rich sources of carbohydrates are corn, beans, millet, green peas, pumpkin, yams, etc.

Increase your intake of foods rich in folic acid. If you are pregnant, the wheat free diet may be bad for you due to folic acid deficiency. However, if you increase your intake of foods that are rich in folic acid aside from wheat, you can still get the right amount of folic acid your body needs even if you are on a wheat free diet. Some foods that are rich in folic acid are spinach; asparagus, legumes as well as you can take folic acid supplements recommended by your doctor.

Use your creativity in baking pastries using wheat-free flours. Without the intake of pastries you love such as cakes, etc. wheat free diet can be boring. But if you use your creativity and bear in mind that there are other types of flour aside from wheat flour, you can bake pastries using these wheat flour alternatives. Non-wheat flours are cassava flour, rice flour, millet flour, soy flour, buckwheat flour, etc. They are not made of wheat and so, you can still reap the benefits of a wheat free diet at the same time, being able to eat pastries.

Always remember that wheat free diet does not necessarily mean gluten-free diet. If you want to rid yourself of celiac disease which is why you are going on a wheat free diet, remember that it's not naturally a gluten-free diet. You can still trigger your celiac disease if you consume non-wheat food items that are rich in gluten. So, in order to get the benefits of a wheat fee diet without compromising your gluten-free diet needs, meditate whether you are dieting wheat free for celiac diseases recovery or simply to lose weight, etc. If it is for your celiac disease, then you must altogether avoid gluten foods and not just wheat free foods.

Consult your doctor. If there is anybody who knows about the type of diet you need, it is your doctor. Remember that the wheat free diet may or may not be good for you depending on your health condition and your purpose as well as there may also be other advice and instructions needed before you start your wheat free diet. This way, it helps when you consult your doctor first to ensure that you will only be reaping wheat free diet benefits as well as totally avoid undesirable effects.

The benefits of a wheat free diet can be very tempting especially if it goes along with your purpose. And since unlike other types of diet, it is not that restrictive, it's not a surprise why a lot of dieters go for this type of diet. As long as you know the foods to avoid, the foods to include and as long as you create a wheat free diet meal plan already, you can start going wheat free right away.

But if you want to truly rake in the wheat free diet benefits and truly bash side effects, it is just right to get to know what the possible side effects are so you can avoid them. It is also advised to abide by some tips towards a successful wheat free diet. Overall, a wheat free diet can be the best solution for whatever purpose you have when it comes to health and fitness.

Thank You Page

I want to personally thank you for reading my book. I hope you found information in this book useful and I would be very grateful if you could leave your honest review about this book. I certainly want to thank you in advance for doing this.

www.ingramcontent.com/pod-product-compliance
Lightning Source LLC
Chambersburg PA
CBHW070524290526
45790CB00003B/1288